Frequently Asked Questions

all about
saw palmetto
and prostate health

MICHAEL JANSON, MD

AVERY PUBLISHING GROUP
Garden City Park • New York

D1736340

The information contained in this book is based upon the research and personal and professional experiences of the author. It is not intended as a substitute for consulting with your physician or other health care provider. Any attempt to diagnose and treat an illness should be done under the direction of a health care professional.

The publisher does not advocate the use of any particular health care protocol, but believes the information in this book should be available to the public. The publisher and author are not responsible for any adverse effects or consequences resulting from the use of any of the suggestions, preparations, or procedures discussed in this book. Should the reader have any questions concerning the appropriateness of any procedure or preparation mentioned, the author and the publisher strongly suggest consulting a professional health care advisor.

Series cover designer: Eric Macaluso
Cover image courtesy of Steven Foster Group, Inc.

Avery Publishing Group, Inc.
120 Old Broadway, Garden City Park, NY 11040
1-800-548-5757 or visit us at www.averypublishing.com

ISBN: 0-89529-939-9

Printed in the United States of America

10   9   8   7   6   5   4   3   2   1

Contents

Introduction, 5

1. The Prostate Gland in Men's Health, 9

2. Saw Palmetto—The Men's Herb, 27

3. Buying and Using Saw Palmetto, 47

4. Other Steps to a Healthy Prostate, 61

Conclusion, 79

Glossary, 81

References, 85

Suggested Readings, 89

Index, 91

Introduction

If you're a man over the age of 50, odds are that you've experienced some prostate problems. Although your prostate gland is relatively small, its location influences the health of your urinary system and aspects of your sexuality. Common symptoms of enlarged prostate include having to get up in the middle of the night to urinate, not feeling like you've completely emptied yourself, and sometimes dribbling. Yes, prostate problems can be embarrassing—but they can also lead to more serious discomforts and disease.

Yet you don't have to face the prospect of synthetic drugs or surgery—and their unpleasant side effects—to correct prostate disorders. A popular herbal treatment, using saw palmetto, has considerable scientific evidence supporting its benefits in prostate disorders. It's also safe and inexpensive.

Like many physicians, when I finished medical school, I knew very little about nutrition and herbal remedies. Although I did learn the biochemistry of the individual nutrients, I did not have any training in how that fit into dietary habits or how the nutrients could be used as dietary supplements for treatment of different medical conditions. I also had no information about herbs and botanicals, which at one time had been the mainstay of medicine in this country, and still contribute greatly to the medical therapy in many countries.

Meanwhile, in Germany and other countries, a large number of general practitioners use herbs routinely. In the United States, a small percentage of doctors have been using these treatments—including vitamins, minerals, amino acids, essential oils and botanicals—for many years for their patients with great success. Often, these doctors have been the objects of ridicule among their peers. They have also been the objects of disciplinary action by their medical boards, which regulate the practice of medicine in every state. Public demand, fortunately, has been forcing a change in this policy, and creating a more congenial atmosphere for innovative physicians.

With this surge of interest, saw palmetto has become one of the most popular dietary supplements. Many more doctors are now recommending saw palmetto for the treatment of prostate disorders. This is based on its long history of use in folk medicine for treatment of urinary tract disorders, and on the recent research supporting its value. In *All About Saw Palmetto and Prostate Health*, you'll learn about this simple, safe, effective, and cost effective dietary supplement to manage your prostate problems, and possibly avoid medication and surgery.

1.

The Prostate Gland
in Men's Health

Practically everyone has heard of the prostate gland, but not everyone knows exactly what it is or how it is important in health. As men age, it is almost certain that they will become familiar with the details of their prostate gland and possibly have to deal with it as a health problem. The more you know about your prostate, the easier it will be to understand how to help yourself or help your doctor understand the treatments best for you.

Q. What is the prostate gland?

A. The prostate gland is a small organ found only in men. It sits below and behind the bladder and above and in front of the rectum. The prostate consists of a collection of glandular tissue, ducts, mus-

cle tissue, and fibrous tissue. It surrounds the urethra, the tube that allows urine to flow from the
bladder through the penis. The prostate is about the
size of a walnut, weighing about two-thirds of an
ounce, and it produces prostatic fluids that combine
with sperm from the testicles and other secretions to
form semen. These fluids help sperm survive and
improve their ability to travel.

The prostate also has some muscle fibers sur-
rounding the urethra that help with other functions,
including urination. With orgasm, the muscles push
some of the prostate fluid with some of the sperm
from the testicles into the urethra and out through
the penis. Although it is very small, the strategic
location of the prostate leads to far more health
problems and medical care costs than would be pre-
dicted from its size alone. One of the most common
and problematic changes in the prostate results
from its gradual enlargement with age (benign
enlargement, not a cancer). This enlargement eventually leads to compression of the urethra and
restriction of the urine flow. It is called benign prostatic hyperplasia (BPH). In addition to the symptoms of obstruction that enlargement causes (the
mechanical or static component of BPH), the muscles and nerves of the prostate, bladder outlet, and
urethra can contribute to other symptoms.

Q. How common are prostate problems?

A. Prostate problems are very common, indeed. More than 50 percent of men over the age of forty have enlarged prostate glands. By the time they reach eighty years old, 80 to 90 percent of men have enlargement of the prostate. Although surgery to remove some of the prostate tissue is a common procedure for benign enlargement, it is not always necessary. Enlarged prostates lead to about $4 billion of health care expenditures, according to a 1996 study.

There are also other possible problems with the prostate. It can be inflamed as a result of infection with bacteria or other organisms, leading to local aching, and pain and burning on urination. This prostate inflammation, or prostatitis, can be acute or chronic. About one-third of the time, the same symptoms occur with no obvious infectious cause.

The prostate is also subject to cellular changes that lead to cancer, the most common cancer in men. Prostate cancers are often undiagnosed, and only found at autopsy when a man dies from other causes. As with many other cancers, diet may play a significant role in the development of prostate cancer.

Q. What are the symptoms when the prostate becomes enlarged?

A. The symptoms of benign prostatic hyperplasia (BPH) are referred to as either variable or dynamic. The variable symptoms refer to the urgency and frequency of urination. The dynamic symptoms refer to the obstruction or compression of the muscles and nerves of the prostate, bladder outlet, and urethra.

BPH leads to a gradual pinching of the urethra and obstruction of the urine flow. The early variable symptoms may simply start with reduction of the size and force of the urine stream. Young men with normal prostates have a peak urine flow of about two-thirds of an ounce (20 ml) per second or higher. This normally declines with age, but even more so with BPH. With mild BPH, the peak flow is reduced to between 15–20 ml per second. With moderate prostate enlargement, the flow rate drops to 10–15 ml per second, and with severe BPH the peak rate is below 10 ml per second.

The urine flow may be difficult to start, a symptom called "hesitancy." This delay in starting urination usually requires some pushing or straining in order to begin the urine flow. Because the bladder muscles assist in the expulsion of the last bit of urine, if there is obstruction of the urethra the muscles will have a more difficult time emptying the bladder completely. (These muscles compensate by getting stronger, so symptoms may not appear early in the course of BPH.) As a result, there may be some residual urine left in the bladder. This retention of urine gives a sensation of incomplete emptying, another sign of prostate enlargement. As a result of the residual urine, there may be more frequent urination.

One of the most distressing symptoms of BPH is frequent nighttime urination. Often, men with prostate enlargement may have to get up two or three or even up to six or more times at night to try to empty the bladder. This is obviously very disturbing to sleep, which is often already a problem for people as they get older. This nighttime urination results from a combination of residual urine, irritation of the urethra and changes in kidney function.

Q. Are there any other symptoms of BPH?

A. Yes, there are a few, and the standard evaluation of patients with prostate enlargement includes a scoring of symptoms to estimate the severity of the problem. For example, difficulty in postponing urination is called "urgency"—the sense that you have to go and can't wait. Sometimes, the urine flow will stop and have to be started again, sometimes with difficulty, a symptom called "interrupted stream," or "intermittency."

Sometimes there is an urge to urinate even when there is very little urine in the bladder. This may result from a combination of physiologic changes in the urethra, bladder, and prostate. With prostate enlargement, straining to start urination, and increased work of the muscles of the bladder and prostate, there may be irritation of the area where the urethra starts in the bladder, or in the early part of the urethra that runs through the prostate (called, naturally enough, the "prostatic urethra"). This irritation makes the sense of urgency greater, and increases the frequency of urination, unrelated to the volume of urine present. Irritation of the urethra and muscle spasms can cause pain or discomfort on urination. This symptom is called dysuria.

Q. Can the severity of the prostate enlargement be measured?

A. In addition to the examinations that doctors do, they use a combination of the self-reported severity for different symptoms of prostate enlargement to come up with a symptom index. One of these symptom scales is a questionnaire called the Boyarsky Index. Patients evaluate the level of nine symptoms on a scale from zero (not present) to three (most severe) for a maximum symptom score of twenty-seven. This scale and modifications of it have been used for many years. Another scale is called the American Urological Association Symptom Index. It uses six symptoms, rated from zero to five, plus the nighttime urinary frequency. In this scale, a score up to seven is mild, up to eighteen is moderate, and above nineteen is considered severe prostatism.

These and other symptom scores give a quantitative evaluation of the severity of prostate symptoms, and they are used to determine the degree of improvement that any treatment provides.

Q. How do I know if I have a prostate problem?

A. Generally, symptoms appear early in the course of benign prostate enlargement, but they are quite variable and subject to many influences, including the perception of the level of discomfort or the amount of sleep disruption. Even with moderate BPH, the symptoms may be minimal because the bladder muscle can grow to compensate for the obstruction.

After the age of 40, annual prostate exams can be very helpful. A doctor will normally do a digital rectal examination (DRE). Because the back of the prostate lies up against the rectum, a doctor can insert a gloved finger into the anal canal and feel if there is some enlargement. However, the local area around the urethra can be enlarged enough to restrict urine flow without enlargement of the entire gland, so it may not be detected by rectal exam of the back of the prostate.

A doctor can also measure the urine flow rate. Other tests include ultrasound studies and magnetic resonance imaging (MRI). These can provide a kind of "picture" of the prostate, but they usually provide little advantage over the symptom evaluation and digital rectal exam.

Q. How can a doctor distinguish between benign prostate enlargement and cancer?

A. Benign enlargement is more common than cancer, but cancer is certainly common enough to be of concern. The prostate may feel different on the rectal examination, since some cancers produce hard, rough, irregular lumps, or nodules. With benign enlargement the prostate is usually softer, smoother, and more even. However, these distinguishing features on examination may not be present in all cases. For example, the nodules of a cancer may be buried within the prostate and not reachable with the doctor's gloved finger.

The doctor can also order a test for a specific substance found in the blood of patients with prostate cancer. This test is the "prostate specific antigen" or PSA. This test is not a perfect tool to distinguish prostate cancer from benign enlargement or prostatitis, but it can help. PSA is a protein molecule produced by prostate cells. The amount of PSA in the blood rises when prostate cells grow or are inflamed. Cancer cells tend to grow more vigorously than other prostate cells, so the level of PSA is likely to be much higher with prostate cancer than with other conditions, but there is overlap. The PSA will also be higher for a day or two after ejaculation, so it is important to give the doctor this information before the test is interpreted.

Q. Are there other tests that are surer in making the diagnosis?

A. Another test that your doctor can do is an ultrasound of the prostate done through the rectum. Ultrasound tests are common in medicine, and they are not dangerous. They are used all the time in evaluating hidden body structures, and in pregnancy to evaluate the developing fetus. Sound waves are reflected off of tissue, and this gives a picture of the prostate and can indicate its size and the presence of lumps that can't be felt. While this test can add some information, it is usually reserved for patients who already have had a positive test (that is, one that has indicated something wrong).

Finally, a doctor can do a biopsy of the prostate. A biopsy is the taking of a tissue sample from a specific organ. It can be an open biopsy, where the surgeon goes in to expose the organ and cuts a piece of tissue. In many cases opening up the body to get to the organ is not necessary, if the organ is accessible to a needle. With this kind of biopsy, a needle is inserted into the gland and a piece of tissue is taken for microscopic examination. This is possible because of the relatively easy access to the prostate gland through the rectum.

Q. What is the usual treatment for BPH?

A. For many years, the only treatment for benign prostatic hypertrophy was to wait until the symptoms were so bad that they were intolerable or the urinary retention created a more serious medical problem. At that time, surgical removal of the obstructive prostate tissue may be necessary. It may be an open operation, from the outside, like many other surgical procedures. It can also be done through a tube (cystoscope) like the one used to examine the inside of the bladder, placed into the urethra through the penis. This is called a "trans-urethral resection of the prostate" or TURP. TURP is still the main treatment for the more severe situations.

As with most surgical procedures, there may be complications from a TURP. One possible effect is "retrograde ejaculation" where the semen is pushed into the bladder rather than out through the penis. Another is impotence, seen in one out of every ten to twenty patients. Involuntary loss of urine (incontinence) is occasionally a problem. Some men develop a urinary tract infection after the surgery, and a repeat operation is often required (in one out of five or ten patients) for recurrent symptoms.

Q. Are these the only treatments for prostate enlargement?

A. No, there are newer treatments that have been developed more recently that are still being studied but seem very promising as far as surgical procedures go. For example, in the so-called TUNA pro-

cedure, or "trans-urethral needle ablation," small
needles are inserted in the prostate by way of a
catheter and they transmit low level radio waves
that create heat and destroy some prostate cells.

Another treatment is called TUMT, or "trans-urethral microwave therapy," in which microwaves are
used to create heat and destroy prostate tissue.
Neither of these procedures is as effective as a
TURP, but both are safer, less invasive, and have
fewer side effects. They also take less time, are less
expensive, and can be done in a doctor's office, usually with very rapid recovery.

Another procedure is the treatment with a
"TULIP" device, which stands for "trans-urethral
ultrasound-guided laser-induced prostatectomy."
This device also destroys some prostate tissue using
a laser beam that is directed at tissue using ultrasound. Like the above procedures, it has fewer side
effects than conventional surgery. However, any
procedure has some associated risks, and no one
wants surgical procedures if they can avoid them.
No doctor recommends such treatments unless the
symptoms are significant.

Q. Are there any non-surgical treatments?

A. Until recently, most conventional physicians

have not had any treatments to offer to patients with prostate enlargement other than to wait until the symptoms worsened to the level where they required surgery. A few years ago, a new medication called finasteride (trade name Proscar®) was shown to help with prostate symptoms. This medication is not nearly as effective as doctors (and especially patients) had hoped it would be. In addition to the low level of benefit, the drug has some side effects that make it less than desirable.

Among the side effects are loss of libido (a decrease of sexual drive), sexual dysfunction (inability to have or maintain an erection), and abnormal ejaculation. There are also risks of birth defects to a male fetus in a pregnant woman who comes in contact with the drug, either through handling the pill or the semen of a man taking it. Because of these potential side effects, and the inadequate results of the treatment with finasteride, both doctors and patients would like to find other ways to treat BPH to reduce symptoms and delay or eliminate the need for surgery. Finasteride appears to work through its effects on hormones and an enzyme.

Q. What are enzymes?

A. Enzymes are protein molecules that act as catalysts—substances that make chemical reactions go faster. The rate of a reaction is determined by many factors, such as heat and the mixture of substances that are reacting. In biological systems, the heat has to be very controlled, so reactions need to be pushed along without excessive heat that might damage cells. This is the role of enzyme catalysts. Enzymes work with other substances, such as minerals and vitamins to push these reactions. Many vitamins are called coenzymes because of their role in helping enzymes work.

Well-known examples of enzymes are the digestive enzymes, produced in the stomach and the pancreas, which work with stomach acids to break down foods. Enzymes also control the reactions that lead to the production of hormones and those involved in the breakdown of hormones after they are used.

Q. What are hormones?

A. Hormones are regulatory substances produced by endocrine glands—these are glands that deliver their output directly into the bloodstream. This is unlike other glands, such as sweat glands or salivary glands, the products of which do not go into the blood. Adrenaline is a well-known example of a hormone. It is produced by the adrenal glands in response to acute stress. Cortisone is another example of a hormone, produce by a different part of the adrenal glands. The pancreas produces insulin, a hormone that regulates blood sugar levels. The thyroid is another endocrine gland. Thyroid hormones regulate metabolic rate, or how fast your body burns energy.

The master endocrine gland is the pituitary at the base of the brain, which produces substances that regulate other glands as well as some hormones that have direct effects on different bodily functions. Among other hormones, the pituitary regulates the amounts of male and female hormones that the body produces. Testosterone and estrogens are examples of male and female sex hormones.

Q. How does finasteride work on hormones?

A. The male sex hormones, or androgens, are primarily testosterone and a derivative called dihydrotestosterone (DHT). DHT is produced from testosterone with the help of an enzyme called 5-alpha reductase. This enzyme is blocked by the drug finasteride. Research suggests that the presence of high levels of DHT promote enlargement of the prostate.

In addition, the female hormone estradiol (one of the estrogens) acts together with DHT in dogs to increase prostate growth, and may also do so in men. (Both men and women have some level of both the male and female hormones, but the balance is different.) Another enzyme, aromatase, converts some of the circulating testosterone into estradiol. Estradiol appears to influence the muscle tissue of the prostate more than the glandular cells, and thus may contribute more to the dynamic symptoms of prostate enlargement than DHT does. Finasteride does not work on the production of estrogen, but there is speculation that blocking DHT production may lead to more estrogen production. This would not be a desirable effect, and may be a reason that finasteride does not work as well as we would like.

Q. What causes the prostate to enlarge?

A. We don't really clearly understand the cause of benign prostate enlargement. We do know that it happens with aging and requires the presence of male hormones, specifically DHT. Men who have had their testicles removed do not develop benign prostatic hyperplasia. We do know that hormonal therapy in dogs that increases the levels of DHT leads to enlargement of the prostate similar to BPH.

In addition, as men age, the level of estradiol in the body increases. In dogs, estradiol works with DHT to induce prostate growth. This is a result of an increase of the amount of receptors in the prostate tissue. If this happens in humans also, it might explain the increase in prostate size with aging.

Lifestyle choices may also play a role, and improper nutrition—specific dietary deficiencies or excesses—may contribute to prostate enlargement. It is also possible that specific foods may contribute to the cause or prevention of prostate enlargement.

Q. Are there any other treatments that doctors usually use?

A. Doctors may prescribe another drug that helps with the dynamic symptoms of prostate enlargement. This drug terazosin (Hytrin®) has been used for high blood pressure because it relaxes the muscles of the blood vessels, allowing them to open and reduce the pressure in the circulation. It is one of a class of drugs called alpha-blockers. The muscles of the prostate and urethra contract in response to hormones that stimulate their "alpha receptors." These are receptors of hormone messages that respond to adrenal type hormones or drugs. Drugs that block these receptors help reduce the symptoms of prostate enlargement and improve urine flow rates by relaxing these muscles.

Q. How well does terazosin work?

A. Terazosin works to improve urine flow but does not affect the size of the prostate. Unfortunately, as with most medications there are some potential side effects from terazosin. Because it is also a blood pressure medication, it may cause you to have low blood pressure, causing dizziness when you stand up or move quickly. It can also cause fatigue, sleepiness, dizziness, and impotence. Another possible problem is nasal congestion and runny nose. One major caution is that the first dose of terazosin may cause very low blood pressure and fainting in the first few days of taking it. If you also have high blood pressure, you may have other side effects.

2.

Saw Palmetto— The Men's Herb

Dietary supplements, including herbs and botanicals, are becoming more popular as treatments for common medical conditions, partly because they usually have the advantage of being safer, more cost effective, and less invasive over drugs and surgery. There are supplements for the heart, the liver, the brain, as well as for diabetes, arthritis, headaches, and many other conditions. Saw palmetto is one that is proving to be quite effective for prostate problems.

Q. Why should I consider taking saw palmetto?

A. Most men will have to consider dealing with their own prostate as they age. If it does become a problem for you, you have the choices outlined in the previous chapter, or you may wish to choose an alternative that has numerous advantages over the drugs and surgery that are the typical treatments. It is no secret that most people would prefer to avoid surgery if possible, especially men who have to contemplate surgery on their prostate gland.

Saw palmetto is a safe, effective alternative to these treatments, based on the medical literature, my own experience using it for patients, and the experience of most of my colleagues in nutritional and botanical medicine. It reduces the symptoms of prostate enlargement, and it also helps improve the objective tests of urinary tract function in a large percentage of men with benign prostatic hyperplasia. You might also consider taking saw palmetto as preventive medicine if you are in the age group at risk for BPH.

Q. What is saw palmetto?

A. Saw palmetto (*Serenoa repens*) is a small palm tree, that grows up to 8 to10 feet high, indigenous to the southeastern coastal states of North America. The tree has large, fan-like leaves, and the berries produced by the tree are about the size of a grape, with a deep reddish-black to brown color. These berries have a long history of use in botanical medicine for disorders of the urinary tract, especially by Native Americans.

More recently, extracts from saw palmetto berries have been medically researched in Europe for their benefits in treating disorders of the prostate gland. These oily extracts are fat soluble and are called "liposterolic extracts." Most of the research on saw palmetto comes from France and Germany, where the use of botanical medicines is more accepted and better researched than in the United States. This is slowly changing as North Americans have developed a strong interest in alternatives to drugs and surgery, and have opened their minds to nutrition and dietary supplements, including botanical medicines. Even the *Journal of the American Medical Association* recently published a very positive article on the use of saw palmetto in the treatment of BPH.

Q. What are botanical medicines?

A. When doctors or other healers use plant extracts in medicine, they might use different parts of certain plants. This is commonly called herbal or botanical medicine. Technically, herbs are the leafy or stem parts of the plant, but when used in medicinal treatments the word "herb" can refer to any part of the plant—the leaf, the stem, the fruit, the bark, or the root. Many botanical medicines are at the root of our modern drugs, such as digitalis for the heart, which comes from foxglove, or colchicine for gout. Aspirin is a derivative of a substance that comes from willow bark.

Q. Why would I choose botanical medicine over conventional?

A. The drugs that doctors commonly use for treatment of illness are often quite risky. Side effects are common, and they can be serious. They can lead to hospitalization and even death. It is no wonder that people are looking for safer and more natural remedies for their health problems. Most of the time, botanical medicines are safer than more recently developed medicines, but that does not mean that they are all without risk. Saw palmetto is one of several natural treatments for prostate disorders.

Q. How does saw palmetto fit into the treatment of the prostate?

A. As already mentioned, saw palmetto can relieve the symptoms of BPH. The clinical effects of saw palmetto seem to be even better than the results seen with finasteride, and without the troubling side effects that are sometimes complications of taking the drug. Saw palmetto is an inhibitor of the enzyme 5-alpha reductase (the enzyme that helps produce DHT, which is the steroid that is believed to cause BPH), but it also appears to have other physiological effects. Some of those effects make it appear superior to the medication, especially when combined with the lack of side effects.

For example, saw palmetto extracts inhibit all of the metabolites of testosterone, not just DHT, and works in all of the cells studied. This is unlike finasteride, which only acts on certain cells and only inhibits certain metabolites. Some research suggests that the male hormones act on the epithelial cells (the actual gland tissue) of the prostate, while the estrogenic hormones act on the structural cells, including muscle tissue and other supporting cells. It appears that saw palmetto inhibits both hormonal actions, and thus reduces both the mechanical and the dynamic components of BPH.

Q. Does saw palmetto have any other effects on the prostate?

A. Research shows that there are other physiological effects of saw palmetto that help prostate symptoms, and may help other medical conditions as well. Extracts of saw palmetto inhibit certain substances that lead to inflammation, irritation, and smooth muscle spasms, among other symptoms. These substances are called "prostanoids," because when they were originally discovered it was thought that they came only from tissue related to the prostate gland. Some of these prostanoids promote inflammation and other types decrease inflammation. If an imbalance among the different types develops it may lead to significant health problems.

As the dynamic symptoms of prostate enlargement are influenced by many of the above processes, saw palmetto can help reduce them. Irritation and spasm of the smooth muscles in the prostate and urethra initiate the urgency and frequency of BPH. Medical research confirms that saw palmetto has benefits for BPH beyond its effect on DHT and the size of the prostate. So it appears that if you have prostate symptoms, you can get some of the benefits of both drugs, finasteride and terazosin, from saw palmetto extracts without the risk of potential side effects seen with the drugs.

Q. How does saw palmetto work on the estrogens?

A. As mentioned above, men produce some female hormones called estrogens (although less than women), just as women produce some testosterone. Receptors are the locations where the hormones bind to cells to have their ultimate effects. You can affect the activity of a hormone without changing the amount that is produced if you change the number of receptors or the ability of the hormone to attach to the receptor sites. To complicate matters further, there are also different kinds of binding sites. Rather than inhibiting the production of the estrogen, saw palmetto works on the receptor sites on which the estrogen works. According to medical reports, saw palmetto works on both kinds of estrogen receptor sites to reduce the activity of estradiol. This would serve another function in reducing BPH symptoms, since estrogens work with DHT to promote BPH.

Q. Why do prostate symptoms vary from time to time while the enlargement does not change back and forth?

A. The variation in prostate symptoms is almost certainly a result of the physical component of BPH. Mental state and stress may also contribute to the symptoms. For example, everyone has had the experience of having a strong urge to urinate, but before finding a bathroom the urge has diminished greatly or even disappeared. This is because the signals from the nerves of the urethra and bladder are variable. Stress may increase the sense of urgency, as can even the sound of running water. The spasms of the muscles of the prostate, bladder, and urethra may also initiate symptoms of urgency and lead to more frequent urination. For these reasons, the urge to urinate can come and go even when the amount of urine in the bladder is unchanged, and in spite of the size of the prostate.

In fact, in a large percentage of patients, symptoms improve with no treatment, even though there is no change in the size of the prostate. Because of this great variation, the placebo effect may have a strong influence on prostate symptoms.

Q. What are placebo effects?

A. When doctors do medical research, they are always on the lookout for effects that appear to be due to a treatment but in reality are due to other factors. This is particularly the case when symptoms of an illness are variable and affected by stress or emotions. It is also an important consideration when the signs of an illness are subjective (reported by the patient) rather than objective (measured by a lab test or other equipment). However, even objective testing can be influenced by subjective feelings.

Symptoms are also affected by expectations of the test subject and even the person administering the test. These are the reasons that medical researchers introduce controls to their studies—to find out if the results are due to these expectations. The term placebo comes from the Latin word meaning to please—the patient tries to please the doctor by reporting that their symptoms are better as a result of the doctor's treatment. The symptoms may actually be better, because we know that the brain has a strong influence on the healing process. But the symptoms may not be influenced by the treatment, which is what the study is trying to determine. This is what is meant by the placebo effect.

Q. How do researchers use placebos?

A. When doing a study, doctors will use a "dummy" pill as one of the treatments in half of the patients. The other half will get a real medicine that the doctors are trying to test. The dummy pill (sometimes formerly called a sugar pill) is called the placebo. It should look exactly like the real treatment, and it is supposed to be completely inactive so that the results of the study are not influenced by any physiological effect induced by the pill. The group receiving the placebo is called the control group. The groups should be carefully matched in every other way to increase the validity of the study.

The subjects in the study are not told if they are receiving the placebo or the real medicine. If that is the only hidden information, it is called a single-blind study. If the persons administering the pills also do not know which group is receiving which pill (they are coded for later interpretation), it is called a "double blind" study. In some studies, after a period of time the groups are switched, so the placebo group is now given the real pill and the study group is given the placebo. This is called a crossover study. (There are problems with some crossover studies because the active ingredients may have long-lasting effects and the effects may not start right away, confusing the results and interpretation.) Studies that are not testing a medication or other substance, but some behavior or stress, can also be conducted in a double blind fashion, but with more difficulty.

Q. Why are placebo-controlled studies important for prostate research?

A. As mentioned above, emotional state, stress, and the placebo effect often influence prostate symptoms. Remember that prostate enlargement symptoms have both static and dynamic components. The dynamic component relates to spasm of the local muscles and irritation of the nerves. These are particularly prone to be influenced by the mind. You probably know that when you are nervous your hands might sweat or they might become cold. Such reactions are everyday evidence of the influence of the mind on physical symptoms. You have probably heard of "mind-body" medicine, referring to the harnessing of the power of the mind to promote healing.

Studies that are designed to show that the effect of a particular treatment is due to the treatment itself, rather than the mind-body influence, need placebo controls to allow researchers to draw accurate conclusions. Although such controlled studies are not the only way to learn about the value of a treatment, doctors do like to see them. Fortunately, many nutritional and herbal treatments have controlled studies that support their value. Saw palmetto has been researched in a number of double-blind, placebo-controlled studies. Often, these studies are done outside the United States. Many of them have been done in France, Germany, and Italy.

Q. What kind of research shows that saw palmetto works for the symptoms of prostate enlargement?

A. Quite a few studies show that saw palmetto works, and they have been published in recognized medical journals. These studies consist of human studies, animal studies, and studies of cells in laboratories. Studies in cells are designed to show how a substance works—what are the biochemical and hormonal actions that can explain the results when the substance is given to a person. Studies in cells have shown some of the actions of saw palmetto. Although we are not sure if the effects that we see in cells in the lab are the ones responsible for the actual results when people take saw palmetto, it is likely that they are related.

Q. When were these studies done and what did they show?

A. The first study on humans that I could find was done in 1979. It was done in Germany and described the treatment of seventy-four men with an extract of Sabal serrulata (another name for saw palmetto). In this study they showed that although the objective measurements of the prostate and urine flow did not change, every patient reported a reduction of their symptoms.

Another early study done on humans was a report by a French team done in 1984. These researchers also reported in another journal the favorable results of using saw palmetto in 110 patients with BPH. Since then there have been a number of other studies that showed similar results. One was done in Spain in 1992 and compared saw palmetto with a drug similar to terazosin. The researchers reported that both substances were about equally effective.

A study done in Italy in 1995 showed that saw palmetto was not quite as effective as another drug similar to terazosin, but still resulted in a reduction of symptoms. This is important for doctors and the public to know, because most people would prefer to take a natural substance if it is almost as effective as and has fewer side effects than a prescription drug, especially if it is less expensive.

Q. Are there any other studies?

A. A study in New Zealand showed that there was similar effect from saw palmetto and finasteride. These patients had improvement in both subjective and objective measures. Nighttime urination, daytime frequency of urination, and peak urine flow rates all improved significantly. In two large uncontrolled trials, about ninety percent of patients reported that their symptoms were much better within three months after starting to take saw palmetto.

Some U.S. doctors only trust studies if they were done in the United States. This is not a reasonable prejudice because studies done in Italy, Germany, France, Spain, and elsewhere are as likely to be valid as those done in the United States. However, one study was done in the United States. In 1998, a team from Chicago evaluated saw palmetto for effectiveness in prostate enlargement. They reported on both objective measurements and patients' reports of their symptoms. They found that after six months about half of the patients reported that they had at least a fifty percent improvement in symptoms, even though the researchers could not measure objective improvements in urine flow. In addition, a recent article in the *Journal of the American Medical*

Association reviewed the research on saw palmetto
and prostate health. Although the authors recommended more research, they acknowledged that
saw palmetto appeared effective and safe.

Q. What was the result of the FDA evaluation of saw palmetto?

A. The United States Food and Drug Administration (FDA) evaluated saw palmetto research in
response to a request by one company in the hope
that they would be able to make a health claim for
their product.

It is interesting that the FDA evaluation of saw
palmetto came shortly after the approval of the prescription drug finasteride. They used several of the
studies mentioned above in their analysis. The FDA
published their conclusions in Food Drug Cosmetic
Law Reports with the following explanations. After
noting that the extract appeared to be safe, they
evaluated nighttime urination frequency, urinary
output, and residual urine, as well as patients'
reports on improvement and discomfort on urination. They noted that the urine volume increased
from five to over eight milliliters per second, the
residual volume decreased from ninety-five to fifty-
five milliliters, and the nighttime urinations de-

creased from over three to an average of 1.7 per night. Over ninety-two percent of the patients reported that their symptoms were better.

These changes, the FDA admitted, were statistically significant. However, they went on to say that they did not consider these improvements to be "clinically significant," because the symptoms were not completely cured, even though in every case they were better than the already-approved drug. Over 90 percent of the patients reported they were better with saw palmetto, while only 50 percent did so with finasteride. The urine flow improved 50 percent with saw palmetto compared to only 22 percent with finasteride. With saw palmetto, residual urine volume went down by forty-two milliliters compared to no change with finasteride. *The Physicians' Desk Reference*, a guide to drugs that every physician uses, states that most patients report at least a thirty percent improvement with finasteride. This is less than in any of the studies that I have seen with saw palmetto.

Q. Has the FDA approved the use of saw palmetto for prostate enlargement?

A. The FDA has not approved the use of saw palmetto for the prostate, but this has to be understood in context. It would be very unusual for the FDA to approve any natural substance in the treatment of medical conditions. Their official role is to assure the safety and promote the development of new drugs. In spite of that, many drugs that reach the market are neither safe nor effective, and eventually are pulled from the market for these very reasons (for example, thalidomide and Fen-phen).

The FDA has an apparent bias against natural products like saw palmetto. Even when they do meet the standards, the FDA seems to find some excuse not to approve them. As mentioned above, the FDA found that saw palmetto produced better results than the prostate drug that they had already approved, but they did not approve saw palmetto. The fact that the FDA has not approved saw palmetto in no way detracts from its value.

Q. Are U.S. doctors recommending saw palmetto?

A. Yes and no. I am, but most doctors here are unfamiliar with herbal or nutritional medicine, and do not recommend saw palmetto. However, naturopaths and nutritionally oriented M.D. and D.O. physicians are among those doctors who do have an interest in alternatives to drugs and surgery. For them, saw palmetto is a common recommendation for prostate enlargement. It is one among several treatments that have research support behind them. Conventional doctors are often opposed to using herbal treatments or other dietary supplements. (Of course, once a doctor starts using such treatments, they are no longer considered conventional.) This is not true in many other countries. In Germany, for example, about half of the primary doctors routinely use these treatments. In 1991 in Italy, herbal treatments represented almost 10 percent of all prescriptions for prostate enlargement.

As increasing numbers of doctors are dissatisfied with the available drug treatments, and as patients are demanding more natural remedies, the group of doctors who do use saw palmetto and other natural treatments is expanding.

Q. How quickly does saw palmetto work for prostate symptoms?

A. Although some patients will report symptom relief sooner, typically a man needs to take saw palmetto for one to three months before significant results can be expected. In some studies, it appears that results are even better if patients continue taking the saw palmetto for six months or more. In the study done in Chicago, one-fifth of patients were better after two months, one-third were better after four months, and nearly half were better after six months. That is when they ended the study, so we don't know if their patients would have had even further improvement with longer treatment.

Q. What is your clinical experience with saw palmetto?

A. I have been treating patients with saw palmetto for a number of years now. In my experience, it is most common for patients to report that their symptoms have improved, usually within two to three months, but sometimes sooner, even within a week or two. Occasionally, patients tell me that their symptoms persist, and it takes much longer for them to see improvement, or they need a higher dose.

Very few patients do not respond to the treatment with saw palmetto, even at the higher dose. For those patients I recommend additional supplements as you will see later. I have been very impressed with the success of this treatment, and I have seen almost no side effects from it, and no serious side effects. As I myself am over fifty years old, I am taking saw palmetto even though I have never had any symptoms of prostate enlargement and have no evidence of it. I am doing this as preventive medicine.

3.

Buying and Using
Saw Palmetto

J ust learning about a supplement is not enough
if you really want to use it for your health. You
really need to know how to take it, the precau-
tions (if any), what dose to use, and how it is
available. You also need to know what to look
for in products, so you are sure to get what is
likely to be most effective for you. I always give
my patients specific instructions, and you need
the same information.

Q. When should I take saw palmetto?

A. There is no special time that will make saw palmetto more or less effective. The most convenient
times to take dietary supplements are with your
breakfast and dinner. Taking supplements with
meals usually helps to avoid any digestive upset
that occasionally occurs with concentrated food

products. Also, there are usually some oils in foods, and these may help with the absorption of the fatty substances in saw palmetto. Most of the researchers have used 160 mg two or three times per day.

You could take your entire daily dose at once, although I usually recommend dividing the dose. However, trying to take it more than twice a day often results in forgetting the other doses, and a supplement that you don't take is going to be totally ineffective. If you don't eat breakfast (although it is a good idea to do so), you can take saw palmetto with lunch and dinner, just as other supplements, or you could take it all in the evening.

Q. What is the correct dose of saw palmetto?

A. The typical dose that is recommended for most men with prostatic enlargement is 160 mg of the standardized extract twice a day. The standardized liposterolic extract of saw palmetto contains 85 to 95 percent sterols and fatty acids. Most of the research is done with this 320-mg daily dose. Some men might benefit from higher doses if the usual dose is not effective. Responses are always variable with any medical treatment, and we have to be prepared to make adjustments for individuals.

I had one eighty-seven-year-old patient who began taking saw palmetto at the 320-mg daily dose, and reported only minimal and sporadic success in relieving symptoms. After almost three years of disappointment, before giving up he decided to take a higher dose for a time. He took twice the usual dose, and after a month reported that the symptoms were almost completely controlled. From a nighttime frequency of three to four urinations, he now only has to get up once or sometimes not at all. He is staying on 320 mg twice a day.

Q. What forms of saw palmetto are available?

A. As with many botanical and herbal treatments, many different preparations are available. There are whole berries, powders made from whole berries, liquid extracts such as tinctures, concentrates, extracts, and "standardized" extracts. It is likely that almost any of the preparations will have some benefit, as long as they honestly contain what is claimed on the label. However, the dose needed to be effective may vary greatly from one brand to another and from one form to another.

For some botanicals, standardized extracts are put into liquid form. Tinctures are extracts in a base of alcohol. You usually take a dropperful or two twice a day, unless otherwise instructed on the label. Some liquid extracts are in a glycerine base for people who prefer to avoid any alcohol. Liquid extracts can be effective if you take enough for your needs.

It is likely that the dose of the berry powders will be far greater than that of the extracts, and it appears that the form most likely to be effective is the standardized extract. However, these are not the only products on the market, and you have to find what works for you. The powders and the standardized extracts may both be available in either tablets or capsules. Some people find capsules easier to swallow, but manufacturers can fit more product into a tablet because they are compressed, and therefore smaller than the comparable dose in a capsule. Most of the time I have seen them in capsules. Read the dose carefully, as some products contain less than the usual 160 mg per pill.

Q. What are standardized extracts?

A. As our knowledge of botanical medicines advances, we are learning to identify the active substances in them that are therapeutic. We are able to research botanicals more easily if we can be sure that the amount of the active substance is consistent from batch to batch. Standardization means that the presumed active principles are always present in approximately the same amount. There is always the chance that other beneficial compounds may be ignored in extracting the supposed active substances.

Most of the recent research on botanical medicines has been done with standardized extracts. Remember, however, that before there were standardized extracts, herbs had been used therapeutically for many centuries, and simple herbal preparations are still of value. If you want the most reliable form of an herb, it is probably best to choose the standardized extracts. Most of them apparently have not only higher levels of the known active compounds, but also higher levels of most of the other potentially active substances.

Q. How do I know if I am getting the right product?

A. If a product contains standardized extract, it should say so on the label. It should also specify that it is standardized to contain "85–95 percent liposterols" right on the ingredient label. If it says simply "extract" or "concentrate" or any other wording, it is probably not the standardized extract. This does not mean that you may not get some value from it, only that it has not been as extensively studied in the recent medical research. Most of the pills on the market contain 120 or 160 mg, so you can take two or three to get the recommended amount.

It is also a good idea to look at the price for a few products (being certain that the doses are comparable). Occasionally, a product will be misbranded, and not contain what the label says. Often these products are less expensive than others. If you compare prices at several health food stores for different brands, and perhaps some mail-order sources of quality brands, you should have some idea of the usual price range for saw palmetto (and similarly for any other health product that you buy). If a product is far above or below the average price, you should be suspicious—on the high end, that you are not receiving value for your money, and on the low end, that you are not getting the right product. (Occasionally you can find good quality brands on special sale at a very good price, but that is usually a temporary deal.)

Q. How long do you have to continue taking saw palmetto?

A. If saw palmetto is working for you, it is likely

that you will have to continue taking it indefinitely. Prostate enlargement is a progressive condition, and it is probable that if you stop taking the treatment, the condition will gradually return. For some of the symptoms, the effect is short term, and they may come back within a short time after you discontinue taking saw palmetto.

We don't have any extended long-term studies that show what happens after someone improves with saw palmetto supplements and then stops taking it. The hormone changes from saw palmetto are likely to continue only for a short time after discontinuing the treatment. Because there are no side effects, it is probably best to continue taking saw palmetto to maintain prostate health and control the symptoms of BPH.

Q. Do the effects wear off if I continue taking it too long?

A. No, none of the evidence suggests this so far. In studies lasting up to twelve months, the improvement in symptoms is maintained and there is no "tolerance" to the herb, meaning that the dose needed to maintain the benefits does not have to be increased. In fact it appears that for some patients the benefits continue to increase during the entire duration of the longer studies. Again, increasing numbers of patients reported improvement if they continued taking the saw palmetto for longer times even at the same dose. I have seen no studies that are extended beyond one year. It seems that from the available research and my own clinical experience, as well as that of my colleagues, that the effects of saw palmetto last well beyond the duration of the studies.

Q. Are there any side effects from saw palmetto?

A. From all the evidence we have, there are almost no side effects from saw palmetto, even in the higher doses. Of course, any substance, even water, given in extremely large quantities may have some negative effects, so it is probably best to stay within the recommended range or even up to double that amount. In the reports that are available, up to 5 percent of patients may report minor side effects, but usually not enough to stop taking the saw palmetto. Often these problems are only minor indigestion, and it usually does not persist. I have only had a few patients report that they had some side effects such as digestive upset, and it was never clearly related to the saw palmetto.

Q. Are there any drugs I cannot take in combination with saw palmetto?

A. There are no contraindications to saw palmetto (medical language for special medical situations in which you should not take a substance). There are also no known negative interactions with drugs or other dietary supplements. In fact, there are other dietary supplements and natural treatments that may help relieve the symptoms of prostate enlargement, and these often enhance the action of the saw palmetto.

Q. Can you take saw palmetto at any age?

A. Yes. If you are under forty years old, unless there is a specific reason to take saw palmetto, I see no reason to recommend it. However, it does not interfere with stamina or endurance and it will not affect your exercise program. The same is true for older people, and as with many herbs and dietary supplements, the unexpected effects are usually beneficial.

In the case of saw palmetto, it may have other benefits for the urinary tract, and it has a history of use for treating inflammation and respiratory symptoms. It has also been used as a mild sedative.

Q. Will saw palmetto interfere with my sleeping pills?

A. No, it won't interfere, and it may even help them work. One of the reasons older men have problems sleeping at night is that prostate enlargement wakes them up frequently to urinate. One of the benefits of taking saw palmetto is that it reduces the frequency of nighttime urination. This in itself may lead to better sleep, and reduce the need for sleeping pills. If the medication is prescribed, there are other considerations.

It is not a good idea to stop taking any medication that has been prescribed without first checking with your doctor. However, if your sleeping does improve after taking saw palmetto, you might consider asking your doctor if you can reduce your medication. Sometimes medications are prescribed for more than one reason, but sleeping pills are usually just for sleep. Doctors sometimes tell patients that a pill is to help them sleep, but it is really for something else and the doctor hopes it will also help sleep. For example, drugs that improve heart function may make it easier to sleep, so be sure you know what you are taking and why before making changes.

Q. I don't have BPH, but I am forty-nine years old. Should I take it anyway?

A. Research studies have not examined the question of whether saw palmetto is valuable as a preventive for prostate problems. Because of its effects on the androgen hormones, it would seem that it should be helpful as prevention by reducing DHT, and some benefit might come from its anti-estrogenic effects. Since you will incur no risk from taking saw palmetto, it is probably a good idea to consider using it as preventive medicine. It does not cost very much so that should not be an obstacle, and again, there are no significant side effects.

The high numbers of men who eventually do have prostate enlargement argue in favor of doing everything possible to prevent it. They are especially adamant about prevention as they pass their fiftieth birthdays, so starting to take saw palmetto in your forties is not unreasonable.

Q. If I am taking saw palmetto, is there any danger to my wife?

A. The drug finasteride (Proscar®) has a history of

some possible problems for women who contact the active ingredient even if they are not themselves taking the drug. For example, if a woman gets pregnant while her partner is taking finasteride, or if she contacts the contents of the pills, she may absorb enough to lead to birth defects in male fetuses in the urinary or genital organs. This may have given some people concern about saw palmetto.

However, there appears to be no risk to male offspring if women who are pregnant come in contact with saw palmetto. Its effects on the hormones and enzymes do not seem to translate to side effects even during pregnancy. Neither finasteride nor saw palmetto has any evidence of side effects directly to a woman who contacts them. In fact, saw palmetto has some possible uses in women as a treatment for some urinary tract conditions.

Q. Is saw palmetto valuable for women in any way?

A. All of the research on saw palmetto that I have seen is on its value for prostate symptoms. However, there is some history of its use in treating urinary tract disorders in both men and women. Saw palmetto has anti-inflammatory properties, and so might well help with the symptoms of urinary tract infections—cystitis and urethritis—such as painful urination. It is not an antibiotic, so it would only help the symptoms, not help eliminate the infection (there are other herbs that help with the infection, such as echinacea and cranberry, as well as drugs).

Saw palmetto may also help women with painful menstrual periods. It may relieve the spasms and cramps that often accompany periods. Although these effects are not well documented, it may be that the effects on estrogen and testosterone hormones might contribute to these benefits.

4.

Other Steps to a Healthy Prostate

Saw palmetto is only one of many dietary supplements that may help the prostate, and it is only part of a comprehensive program for prostate health. A complete program must consider diet, other lifestyle issues, and prevention of disorders of the prostate other than benign enlargement, such as cancer.

Q. Is pygeum the same as saw palmetto?

A. No, pygeum is another natural treatment for the prostate. Its actual name is *Pygeum africanum*, an extract of an African tree bark. It is a botanical that helps relieve prostate symptoms, and it has some research to prove it. In one study, although there were no changes in hormone levels in the blood of patients who took pygeum, all of the evaluations showed improvement in the urinary symptoms and reduction in the swelling of the prostate around the urethra.

In another study, carried out in several centers in France, Germany, and Austria, the researchers found similar results with highly significant improvement in BPH symptoms. The number of nighttime urinations, the residual urine volume, and the urine flow rates all improved, and as in the other studies there were only a few minor side effects.

In yet another study with a placebo control, the researchers showed that although many of the patients improved with the placebo, there were significantly more that did well with the pygeum extract. The improvements were seen in the ease of starting urination, the frequency of nighttime urinations, and in the sensation of incomplete emptying of the bladder.

All of the studies indicate that there are only few and minor side effects from pygeum. This is similar to other natural remedies for the prostate, although some of the patients experienced digestive upset. A comparison of saw palmetto and pygeum in one study showed that both were effective, but saw palmetto was somewhat better. The usual dose of *Pygeum africanum* is 25 to 50 mg of the standardized extract taken twice a day.

Q. Can you take saw palmetto and pygeum together?

A. Yes, this is a common approach to the natural treatment of prostate enlargement. Unlike the situation with many medications, dietary supplements often work well together. In most medical treatments, doctors and patients are looking for some sort of "magic bullet" that will, by itself, cure a problem with few and minor side effects. This is not usually the case in treatments that use both nutrition and dietary supplements. Because nutrients work together in all cells, it is a good idea to combine different treatments unless there is a specific negative interaction. There are no negative interactions when you take saw palmetto and pygeum together.

Although there are only a few studies where several treatments are combined, they have usually shown that different supplements enhance the actions of the others. There are several products available in the health food stores that are combinations of the herbs and nutrients that help the prostate. It may be possible to take a lower dose of each of the supplements that help the prostate if they are taken in combination.

Q. What are the other herbs that help the prostate?

A. Studies with extract of the stinging nettle plant have shown that it reduces prostate symptoms of prostate problems. Nettle may work by its effect on the hormone DHT. It reduces the ability of DHT to bind to the sites where it is active. This results in less activity of the hormone even though the amount remains unchanged.

Nettle extracts appear to enhance the action of pygeum and saw palmetto in studies in which it is combined with either of them. Although stinging nettles get their name from the stinging hairs on their stems and leaves, the extracts do not have an irritant effect. Nettle has been used as a food, and cooking eliminates its irritant properties. In fact, nettle extract has an anti-inflammatory effect and it reduces allergy symptoms, among its other beneficial actions. The typical dose of nettle is 150 to 300 mg twice a day, but for allergies a dose of 300 mg every three to four hours is sometimes recommended.

Q. What other natural treatments are doctors using?

A. For many years, before saw palmetto or pygeum were commonly available as therapeutic supplements, nutritionally-oriented doctors did use other natural remedies for prostate enlargement with some success. One of the most widely used supplements for the prostate has been high doses of the trace mineral zinc. Zinc is important for many different physiological functions, such as the sense of taste and smell, wound healing, immunity, antioxidant activity, and in management of the common cold.

Zinc is particularly important for the normal functioning of the prostate. The prostate gland is very rich in zinc, containing far more than any other organ. It influences the hormones in the prostate, and like saw palmetto can reduce the activity of the enzyme 5-alpha reductase. Small amounts of zinc are necessary for the activity of the enzyme, but higher levels appear to inhibit it.

It is also known that zinc levels are low in those patients with both benign enlargement of the prostate and prostate cancer. Physicians have recommended zinc in doses up to 150 mg per day for prostate enlargement. Recently, recommendations are to take doses of zinc in the range of 30 to 60 mg, and to take it with copper to avoid an imbalance. This lower dose appears to be adequate when you also take other therapeutic supplements that help the prostate.

Q. Do other nutrients help treat prostate enlargement?

A. Yes, there are numerous supplements that help the prostate, partly because they have a direct effect on the prostate tissues, an indirect effect on hormone balance, or effects on other nutrients. For example, vitamin B_6, or pyridoxine, can help the absorption of zinc. Pyridoxine also helps to reduce the production of another hormone called prolactin. Prolactin is produced in the pituitary gland, and it stimulates milk production in lactating women. It also has an effect on the prostate. Prolactin promotes DHT production, and as a consequence it can stimulate prostate tissue growth. Reducing prolactin levels can help reduce the overgrowth of prostate tissue. Typical doses of pyridoxine are in the range of 50 to 200 mg per day. Very high doses, in excess of 500 to 2,000 mg, have on occasion been associated with some neurological symptoms, so it is wise to stay away from the highest doses.

Magnesium may be very important for symptoms of prostate enlargement, particularly the dynamic symptoms that depend on the muscles of the urethra, bladder, and prostate tissue. Magnesium helps to relax these muscles. It is also important to take magnesium when you are taking extra vitamin B_6, because it helps to balance this nutrient. Typical doses of magnesium are from 300 to 1,000 mg daily. I usually recommend magnesium aspartate, one of many available forms. Although most magnesium supplements will work, this one is particularly well absorbed.

Q. Do amino acids affect prostate health?

A. Amino acids are the building blocks of proteins. They get their name from a nitrogen-hydrogen combination called an amine, or amino group. There are eight essential amino acids—the kind you must get from your diet because your body cannot manufacture them.

Most people get enough of the amino acids that they need from the protein that they eat. In fact, most Americans get too much protein, especially animal protein, so they have an abundance of amino acids. Most of the amino acids from foods go into the manufacture of the different proteins of the body, or they are burned for energy, and any excess is converted to fat.

Several reports suggest the value of certain amino acids in the treatment of prostate enlargement. The amino acids glycine, alanine, and glutamic acid were shown to reduce prostate symptoms in seventy to ninety percent of the subjects in a study, depending on which symptom was being evaluated.

When used for treatment, you cannot depend on food sources because other amino acids present in protein drown out the therapeutic ones. You need to take supplements. The daily amounts that are recommended vary from 50 to 200 mg of alanine, 200 to 400 mg of glycine, and 200 to 1,000 mg of glutamic acid.

Q. Do fats play a role in prostate enlargement?

A. Yes, fats and oils can play a very important role in maintaining prostate health or in causing problems with the prostate, depending on the kind of fat, the balance in your diet, and supplements. It is well known that too much fat or the wrong kind of fat in the diet is hazardous to your health in many ways. It is especially a problem when they are animal fats, or if the oils are hydrogenated (such as in margarine and shortening), or heavily processed (such as commercial vegetable oils). Heating any oils during cooking increases the damage to the fat by oxidizing them, creating dangerous byproducts. Although polyunsaturated oils were heavily promoted for a time, they are exactly the ones that have the greatest likelihood of being oxidized by heat and light, and they increase the risk of cancer of many organs.

Most people have too much fat in their diets, but they don't have enough of the essential fatty acids (those that are required in the diet). The right amounts of the essential fatty acids are specifically valuable for prostate health. Research suggests that men with BPH are deficient in the essential fatty acids and that supplements can help. I often recommend a combination of unrefined flaxseed oil for the omega-3 oils (one of the two essential fatty acids) and evening primrose oil or borage oil for the gamma-linolenic acid (GLA) as the omega-6 oil source. Typically, the dose of flaxseed oil is one to two tablespoons per day, and the dose of GLA is 240 mg (equivalent to one capsule of borage oil or six evening primrose oil capsules). Certain fish, such as salmon and sardines, also contain an omega-3 oil called EPA. This oil is also available as a supplement in capsules.

Q. Do any other dietary habits play a role in prostate health?

A. As with almost every disease, lifestyle choices play a role in prevention and treatment of prostate disorders. This is especially true for prevention of prostate cancer, but may also play an important role in prostate enlargement.

Try to choose a diet rich in vegetables, fresh fruits, whole grains, and beans. The more colorful the vegetable or fruit the more likely it is to contain healthful nutrients. Eating meat has been shown to dramatically increase the risk of getting prostate cancer. A vegetarian diet is healthier in many ways than one that includes meat. Avoid adding much oil of any kind to the diet, although olive oil may not cause a problem. Other oils and fats may be a serious risk, and in countries where the fat intake is low, there is a low incidence of prostate cancer. (Black Africans have a low incidence of prostate cancer and a low fat diet, while African Americans have a high incidence of prostate cancer and a high fat intake.) These food selections provide a diet that is high in fiber, and low in fat.

Read ingredient labels carefully and avoid foods that contain added sugar and artificial and synthetic additives, such as flavorings, colors, sweeteners, and preservatives. These add nothing to enhance health and are usually present only in heavily processed foods that you don't need in your diet anyway.

Avoid caffeine and alcohol as much as possible. Caffeine has been associated with fibrocystic disease of the breast, and since the breast contains glandular and fibrous tissue like the prostate, it is possible that caffeine may cause problems for the prostate also. Alcohol affects the hormones that play a role in prostate enlargement, and it is best to keep alcohol intake low.

Q. Are there specific foods that may help prevent prostate cancer?

A. Yes, several foods are more specific than the general guidelines above. Include some soybean products in your diet, such as tofu or soy milk. Natural hormone-like substances in soy (called phytoestrogens) help to prevent cancer of the prostate and many other organs. Other forms of soy products are tempeh, a fermented soybean cake common in Indonesia, and soy protein powders that can be added to fruit smoothies, other blender drinks, or even vegetable stews.

Whole grains have also been shown to decrease

cancer risks. In population studies, those who have the highest intake of whole grains have a lower incidence of cancer for almost every cancer studied, including prostate. This means it is important to include whole grains in the diet, such as brown rice, oatmeal, whole wheat, millet, barley, corn, rye, and several others.

Q. What specific nutrients can help?

A. Lycopene is in the carotene family of vitamins (beta-carotene is the best-known carotenoid, but there are many other nutritious carotenoids). Lycopene is found in tomatoes, and it is also available as a supplement. Research shows that eating tomatoes can reduce the risk of prostate cancer, most likely because of the lycopene content. Men whose diets are high in lycopene have a lower chance of getting prostate cancer than men with lower levels of lycopene intake. Any tomato product is beneficial, from fresh tomatoes, to tomato sauce to tomato juice, or you can take lycopene supplements.

Garlic contains a number of substances that are protective. Whether taken as a food or as a supplement, it is associated with a lower chance of getting prostate cancer. Garlic is commonly available in a deodorized supplement for those who don't like garlic or don't wish to smell it every day. (I personally like it a lot, and eat it often, and it is a common ingredient in many of the ethnic foods that I enjoy.) Supplements of deodorized garlic commonly contain about 500 mg of concentrated extract. You might take two to four of these a day if you are not eating garlic regularly.

Selenium is a trace mineral that protects against many cancers. It is low in many peoples' diets, but it is readily available as an inexpensive supplement. Typical supplemental doses range from 100 to 400 mcg (micrograms) a day.

Q. Can exercise help improve prostate health?

A. As with almost any health issue, it is important to get regular exercise, such as walking, jogging, skiing, skating, bicycling, or using exercising machines. Specific exercises that help urinary control consist of contracting the muscles around the rectal area as though trying to stop urination or a bowel movement. These are known as Kegel exercises, and doing them many times a day may help in bladder control.

Try to do at least thirty minutes of exercise most days. When people ask me if they have to exercise every day, I ask them "How often does a gorilla exercise?" The answer, of course, is every time they want to eat or play, which is more than once a day. This may be too much to fit into your schedule (gorillas don't have to work) but there is consensus that exercising at least four to six times a week is beneficial. It has even been associated with a decreased risk of cancer as well as heart disease.

If you have not been doing exercise regularly, start with just ten or fifteen minutes of walking and increasing your time by a few minutes a week. It is easy to determine how fast to go, because you should not get out of breath during the exercise, but you should work up a sweat by the time you get to thirty minutes. You don't need a formal exercise program if you keep very active, such as by gardening, mowing the lawn, walking or bicycling on your errands, and taking stairs instead of elevators when possible.

Q. Does stress or other lifestyle issues play a role in prostate health?

A. The placebo effect demonstrates that most illnesses are influenced by emotional state, thought processes, and expectations. They lead to both the feeling of improvement and actual measurable improvement. If such things can be helpful in managing illness, it is clear that they can also be involved in causing or worsening symptoms. Stress increases general health risks, and leads to increased output of the adrenal hormones. It also leads to increased metabolism, and damaging oxidation byproducts. Practicing a stress reduction technique can be very helpful with general health and reducing cancer risks.

Try to do some relaxation exercises such as breathing exercises, yoga, stretching, or simply closing your eyes and imagining your favorite place for about three or four minutes five or six times a day. You might consider reading about meditation or getting some help learning how to do it if that is your preference. Whatever relaxation method works for you is fine.

Q. Does smoking affect prostate health?

A. I can't say enough about the dangers of tobacco smoke, even second-hand smoke to which most of us are exposed. It is probably one of the most dangerous substances to which humans expose themselves voluntarily. It leads to many cancers, including cancer of the prostate, and puts a great burden on your normal protective mechanisms. Avoid it.

Q. Will prostate disorders affect my sex life?

A. Benign enlargement of the prostate need not affect your sexual function at all, depending on how severe it is and how much it makes you uncomfortable. It does not affect your libido (sex drive), your ability to have an erection, or your ability to have normal orgasms and ejaculations. If you are taking saw palmetto for enlarged prostate symptoms, it has no side effects, and it has even been used to enhance libido and potency.

If you have infection or inflammation of the prostate that leads to painful or uncomfortable urination, it may temporarily decrease your desire or sexual function. This should clear up after proper treatment of the infection. While being treated, it is a good idea to take dietary supplements that may help reduce the inflammation and speed your recovery from the infection.

Early prostate cancer is also not a problem, but in the later stages or after treatment with surgery, radiation, or drugs, it is more common to see interference with sexual function. This is often not a permanent problem, depending on the treatment. Even after surgery to remove the prostate, most men can have an active sex life. The prostate is not essential to the desire or ability to have sex.

Remember that prostate enlargement is extremely common, it should not interfere with your sexual pleasure, and many natural treatments help to avoid the side effects of drugs and surgery. There is no reason not to feel good about yourself in spite of an enlarged prostate or even prostate cancer. Sexual activity probably helps to maintain the health of the prostate.

Conclusion

Saw palmetto is a part of a comprehensive program to take care of your prostate. Programs like this one can help with almost any health problem, and it gives you some measure of control over your own care. Your doctor may be very willing to participate in this kind of care, because many doctors are becoming aware of the interest of their patients in more natural remedies. If your doctor is unwilling to consider using saw palmetto or other dietary supplements, perhaps you should give him or her a copy of this book.

Consider all of the options no matter what your health problems, and make informed decisions about the kind of care that you want. If you can't find a doctor who will work with you in this form of treatment, you can call the American College for Advancement in Medicine (ACAM) at 800-532-3688 to locate a doctor in your area who is open to innovative treatments. You could also look them up on the internet at http://www.acam.org.

Using natural remedies as part of your comprehensive health care for both treatment and prevention is a positive step in the changing health care picture. Increasing numbers of doctors are becoming aware of these treatments and adding them to their medical skills. An even larger percentage of the American population is doing this, and you would do well to join them.

Glossary

Amino acids. The building blocks of proteins that get their name from a nitrogen-hydrogen combination called an amine that is always a part of the molecule.

Botanical medicine. Any plant-derived medicinal treatment, regardless which part of the plant is used.

BPH. Benign prostatic hyperplasia, or enlargement of the prostate that leads to a pinching off of the urethra, or urinary outflow tract.

DHT. Dihydrotestosterone, a hormone derived from testosterone that is an apparent cause of benign enlargement of the prostate.

DRE. A digital rectal examination, in which a doctor places a gloved finger in the rectum to evaluate the size and shape of the prostate gland.

Dysuria. Pain or discomfort on urination that results from irritation of the urethra and spasms of the bladder and prostate muscles.

Enzymes. Protein molecules that act as catalysts—substances that make biochemical reactions go faster.

Essential fatty acids. The oils that are needed in normal physiology and that you must consume in the diet because your body cannot make them.

Herbal medicine. Any medicinal product derived from the leafy or stem parts of a plant, but also commonly used to refer to any botanical medicine regardless which part of the plant is used.

Hormone. Regulatory substances produced by endocrine glands—glands that deliver their output directly into the bloodstream.

Placebo effect. Any benefit that a patient experiences or is measured by tests that is due to a patient's expectation of improvement from a treatment, rather than from the specific treatment that is being administered.

Prostate. A small organ, found only in men, that sits below and behind the bladder and produces prostatic fluids that combine with sperm from the testicles and other secretions to form semen.

PSA. "Prostate specific antigen," a test for a specific substance found in abnormally high amounts in the blood of patients with prostate cancer.

Pygeum. *Pygeum africanum*, a botanical extract from an African tree bark that helps reduce the symptoms of BPH.

Saw palmetto. A small palm tree with red-brown berries that have been medically researched in Europe and the United States for their benefits in treating disorders of the prostate gland.

Standardized extract. Herbal medicines that contain specific amounts of the most likely active components based on the current state of research, but which also contain other principles of the plant.

Urethra. The urine outflow tract from the bladder through the penis (not to be confused with the ureters, which carry urine from the kidneys to the bladder).

References

Kortt MA, Bootman JL, "The economics of benign prostatic hyperplasia treatment: a literature review." *Clin Ther* (Nov–Dec 1996): 18(6):1227–41.

Flamm J, Kiesswetter H, "An urodynamic study of patients with benign prostatic hypertrophy treated conservatively with phytotherapy or testosterone." *Wien Klin Wochenschr* (Sep 1979) 28;91(18):622–7.

Champault G, Patel JC, Bonnard AM, "A double-blind trial of an extract of the plant Serenoa repens in benign prostatic hyperplasia." *Br J Clin Pharmacol* (Sep 1984): 18(3):461–2.

Champault G, Bonnard AM, et al., "Actualite Therapeutique: The medical treatment of prostatic adenoma." *Ann Urol* (1984): 6: 407–10.

Adriazola Semino M, Lozano Ortega JL, Garcia Cobo E, Tejeda Banez E, Romero Rodriguez F, "Symptomatic treatment of benign hypertrophy of the prostate. Comparative study of prazosin and serenoa repens." *Arch Esp Urol* (Apr 1992): 45(3): 211–3.

Grasso M, Montesano A, Buonaguidi A, et al., "Comparative effects of alfuzosin versus Serenoa repens in the treatment of symptomatic benign prostatic hyperplasia." *Arch Esp Urol* (Jan-Feb 1995): 48(1):97–103.

Plosker GL, Brogden RN, "Serenoa repens (Permixon). A review of its pharmacology and therapeutic efficacy in benign prostatic hyperplasia." *Drugs Aging* (Nov 1996): 9(5):379–95.

Braeckman J, "The extract of Serenoa repens in the treatment of benign prostatic hyperplasia: a multicenter open study." *Curr Ther Res* (1994): 55:776–85.

Schneider HJ, Honold E, Masuhr T, "Treatment of benign prostatic hyperplasia: results of a surveillance study in the practices of urological specialists using a combined plant-based preparation." *Fortsch Med* (1995): 113:37–40.

Gerber GS, Zagaja GP, Bales GT, Chodak GW, Contreras BA, "Saw palmetto (Serenoa repens) in men with lower urinary tract symptoms: effects on urodynamic parameters and voiding symptoms." *Urology* (Jun 1998): 51(6):1003–7.

Food Drug Cosmetic Law Reports, "New Developments," (March 5, 1990) 1427:42,434–41.

Carani C, Salvioli V, Scuteri A, Borelli A, Baldini A, Granata AR, Marrama P, "Urological and sexual evaluation of treatment of benign prostatic disease using Pygeum africanum at high doses." *Arch Ital Urol Nefrol Androl* (Sep 1991): 63(3):341–5.

Barlet A, Albrecht J, Aubert A, et al., "Efficacy of Pygeum africanum extract in the medical therapy of urination disorders due to benign prostatic hyperplasia: evaluation of objective and subjective parameters. A placebo-controlled double-blind multicenter study." *Wien Klin Wochenschr* (Nov 1990): 23;102(22):667–73.

Dufour B, Choquenet C, Revol M, Faure G, Jorest R, "Controlled study of the effects of Pygeum africanum extract on the functional symptoms of prostatic adenoma." *Ann Urol* (Paris) (May 1984): 18(3):193–5.

Krzeski T, Kazon M, Borkowski A, Witeska A, Kuczera J, "Combined extracts of Urtica dioica and Pygeum africanum in the treatment of benign prostatic hyperplasia: double-blind comparison of two doses." *Clin Ther* (Nov-Dec 1993): 15(6):1011–20.

Schneider HJ, Honold E, Masuhr T, "Treatment of benign prostatic hyperplasia. Results of a treatment study with the phytogenic combination of Sabal extract WS 1473 and Urtica extract WS 1031 in urologic specialty practices." *Fortschr Med* (Jan 1995): 30;113(3):37–40.

Habib FK, Hammond GL, Lee IR, et al., "Metal-androgen interrelationships in carcinoma and hyperplasia of the human prostate." *J Endocrinol* (Oct 1976): 71(1):133–41.

Wynder EL, Rose DP, Cohen LA, "Nutrition and prostate cancer: a proposal for dietary intervention." *Nutr Cancer* (1994): 22(1); 1–9.

Chatenoud L, Tavani A, La Vecchia C, Jacobs DR Jr, Negri E, Levi F, Franceschi S, "Whole grain food intake and cancer risk." *Int J Cancer* (Jul 1998): 3;77(1):24–8.

Suggested Readings

Janson, M. *The Vitamin Revolution in Health Care.* Greenville, NH: Arcadia Press, 1996.

Murray, M., Pizzorno, J. *Encyclopedia of Natural Medicine.* Rocklin, CA: Prima Publishing, 1991.

Schachter, M. *The Natural Way to a Healthy Prostate.* New Canaan, CT: Keats Publishing, 1995.

Werbach, M., Murray, M. *Botanical Influences on Illness.* Tarzana, CA: Third Line Press, 1994.

Index

American Urological
    Association
    Symptom Index, 15
Amino acids, 67–68

Benign prostatic hyper-
    plasia (BPH), 10
    cancer and, distin-
        guishing between,
        16–17
    causes of, 24–25
    diagnosing, 15–18
    dietary fat and, 68–69
    measuring severity of,
        14–15
    sexual function and,
        76–77
    symptoms of, 12–14,
        15

treatments for, con-
    ventional, 18–21,
    23–24, 25–26
treatments for, natural.
    See Magnesium;
    Nettle; Pyridoxine;
    Saw Palmetto; Zinc.
Biopsy, 18
Botanical medicines,
    29–30, 50–51
Boyarsky index, 15
BPH. *See* Benign prosta-
    tic hyperplasia.

Cancer of the prostate.
    See Prostate cancer.

DHT. *See*
    Dihydrotestosterone.

Diagnosis of prostate problems, 15–18

Dietary habits, prostate health and, 70–71

Digital rectal examination (DRE), 16

Dihydrotestosterone (DHT), 23, 24, 31, 64, 66

DRE. *See* Digital rectal examination.

Dysuria, 14

Enzymes, 21–22

Estradiol, 24, 25

Estrogen, 24
saw palmetto and, 32–33

Exercise, prostate health and, 73–74

Fatty acids, 68–69

FDA. *See* Food and Drug Administration, saw palmetto and.

Finasteride, 21, 31, 40, 57–58

hormones and, 23–24

5-alpha reductase, 23, 31, 65

Food and Drug Administration (FDA), saw palmetto and, 41–43

Garlic, 72–73

Herbal medicine. *See* Botanical medicines.

Hormones
about, 22–23
finasteride and, 23–24

Intermittency. *See* Interrupted stream.

Interrupted stream, 14

Journal of the American Medical Association, 29, 40–41

Lycopene, 72

Magnesium, 66–67

Magnetic resonance imaging (MRI), 16

MRI. *See* Magnetic resonance imaging.

Nettle, 64

Physicians' Desk Reference, 42

Placebo effect, 34–35, 74. *See also* Placebo-controlled studies.

Placebo-controlled studies
  about, 35–36
  prostate research and, 37–38

Prolactin, 66

Prostanoids, 32

Prostate cancer, 11
  BPH and, distinguishing between, 16–17
  dietary habits and, 70–73
  sexual function and, 76–77

Prostate gland

about, 9–10

cancer of. *See* Prostate cancer.

enlargement of. *See* Benign prostatic hyperplasia.

inflammation of. *See* Prostatitis.

Prostate specific antigen (PSA), 17

Prostatic urethra, 14

Prostatitis, 11

PSA. *See* Prostate specific antigen.

Pygeum, 61–63

Pygeum africanum. *See* Pygeum.

Pyridoxine, 66

Saw palmetto
  about, 28–29
  BPH and, 30–33
  dosage, suggested, 48–49
  drugs, taken with, 55, 56
  estrogens and, 32–33

FDA and, 41–43

forms of, 49–50

how long to take, 52–53

preventative, as a, 57

pygeum, taken with, 63

reasons for taking, 27–28

research on, 38–41

side effects of, 54

symptom relief and, 44–46

when to take, 47–48

women and, 57–59

Selenium, 73

Serona repens. *See* Saw palmetto.

Sexual function, prostate health and, 76–77

Sleeping pills, saw palmetto and, 56

Smoking, prostate health and, 75

Standardized extracts, about, 50–52

Stinging nettle. *See* Nettle.

Stress, prostate health and, 75

Symptoms of BPH, 12–14, 15

reason for variation of, 33–34

Terazosin, 25–26

Testosterone, 23

Trans-urethral microwave therapy (TUMT), 20

Trans-urethral needle ablation (TUNA), 19–20

Trans-urethral resection of the prostate (TURP), 19

Trans-urethral ultrasound-guided laser-induced prostatectomy (TULIP), 20

TULIP. *See* Transurethral ultrasound-guided laser-induced prostatectomy.

TUMT. *See* Trans-
urethral microwave
therapy.
TUNA. *See* Trans-
urethral needle
ablation.
TURP. *See* Trans-
urethral resection
of the prostate.

Ultrasound tests, 17–18
Urethra, 10
Urgency, 13–14

Urinary tract infections,
saw palmetto and,
58–59
Urine flow, 12–13
terazosin and, 26

Vitamin B_6. *See*
Pyridoxine.

Women, saw palmetto
and, 57–59

Zinc, 65